LOSE WEIGHT
SAVE MONEY AND
REALLY REDUCE
GREENHOUSE GASES

Radical Shifts in Military, Electrical, Construction, Transportation, Medical, Agricultural, Entertainment and Economic Systems to End Global Warming, Obesity and Poverty

Stephen Simac

This is the second edition of Lose Weight, Save Money and
Really Reduce Greenhouse Gases
first edition published in 2014

Also by author
The Medical Monopoly Series
Save Trillions with Universal Health Care
Cancer Cathedral: Prevention is the Cure
Mandatory Vaccination - Totalitarian Inoculation

Table of Contents

Introduction

Chapter 1 A Heliocentric Solar System

Chapter 2 Time for New Slogans

Chapter 3 Addiction Creates Necessity

Chapter 4 The Cult of the Military

Chapter 5 Electric Avenue

Chapter 6 Sustainable Castles

Chapter 7 The Velorution

Chapter 8 Put the Lime in the Coconut

Chapter 9 The Fall of Western Civ

Chapter 10 Flickering Blue Tubes

Chapter 11 A Better Future Being Born

Introduction

This is no pyramid scam, even if it sounds suspiciously like one. Most Americans want to lose weight and save some money. Even more so, when it also prevents an environmental disaster that threatens the fate of human society. That's a bonus. This plan will also lower your medical bills, make you smarter and sexier with whiter teeth too. Everyone's a winner.

Unless, of course more urgent desires distract us from the sensible goals presented here to radically reduce Greenhouse Gases (GHG). This book identifies the major sources of human generated GHG contributing to Global Warming, (GW), Climate Change (CC), Extreme Weather Phenomena (EWP) or the latest acronym to explain what's going on with the weather. It reports on available, practical solutions that will drastically reduce emissions and make America cleaner, safer and healthier.

Entire industries depend on pumping GHG out into the atmosphere and oceans without paying for their social and environmental cost. They'd like to keep it that way. It won't be easy to achieve these goals, even if human civilization depends on us doing so because of their influence. However the rewards for individuals and society from really reducing GHG are enormous, aside from benefiting the entire planet. If they actually believe in GW, most Americans want to reduce GHG. Only about half to a third of Americans do believe according to various polls depending on the season. Far fewer are doing more than snapping their fingers while the Titanic sinks.

Belief seems to fluctuate as widely as the weather, despite a relentless PR campaign to convince us of impending doom from GW. Most scientists, media pundits and Democrat politicians are on board, but since many Americans don't trust those authorities to be fair and balanced, this may do more harm than good. The numbers of believers should increase if climate prognostications are correct. Especially those who live near the coast or in a trailer, both particularly susceptible to predicted results from our carbon belching ways.

Americans are addicted to emitting vast quantities of carbon and methane, the two major sources of human created GHG. Reducing our carbon footprint, much less our methane mittens is a hard sell. Our high powered, glamorous society runs on the stuff. Any politician or environmental expert claiming that the American Way Of Life (AWOL), only needs to be tweaked a bit to neutralize our Carbon Bigfootprint is lying. Massive changes will have to be made if we're going to make a halfway decent dent in GHG.

Luckily those changes are affordable and healthier for people and the planet. AWOL is a known cause of poor health, widespread obesity and much of our stress and unhappiness. It's not affordable, much less sustainable. So changing our self destructive habits, while saving the planet seems like a great idea, something that should be easy for people to get onboard. But like any addiction, quitting is never easy and sobriety a long struggle.

That's why legislation to really reduce GHG plays poorly both in the blessed heartland and from coast to coast. Politicians aren't going to be the first on board that train. They'll wait until it's more than half full. We are addicted to fossil fuels to maintain AWOL and seemingly powerless to control our addiction. That's the first step. Get out of Denial. We're not actually helpless, so a higher power isn't necessary. Reality must spur us towards sustainability. The second step is to understand that we've been sold a lifestyle that can't possibly withstand the coming superstorms. We are the little piggies in the straw house, and it ain't strawbale.

Americans burn through one quarter of the world's energy use. We emit an equal percentage of GHG, although we're only 5% of global population. Even our 5% of the planet's children own half the toys. We squander the world's resources because we believe that's what we need to be comfortable, what we've become accustomed to, never really thought deeply about. We could live far healthier, cheaper, cleaner, safer lives and burn a lot less fossil fuel. Those who really want to reduce GHG must coalesce around envisioning the transformation needed in systems we're embedded in. It will be like waking up in The Matrix and choosing a different pill than the one we're being force fed in our sleep.

AWOL, defended so fiercely by our military overseas and legal and economic system at home, is touted as a comfortable yet pleasantly stimulating lifestyle by the advertisers selling it to us. If that's so, then why are almost half of adult Americans suffering from chronic pain from one or more debilitating illnesses or injuries? Pain meds are in every senior's bathroom cabinet while teenagers are snorting their parents' pills to feel better for a short spell. Anti-Depressants are flying out of the pharmacies, prescribed to patients in droves because of AWOL. Maintaining AWOL causes so much stress and costs so much that many Americans have already tumbled off the cliff the rest are headed for.

AWOL has caused us to basically desert our duties as stewards of the environment and our own physical and emotional health. It's guaranteed to put on weight, cause illness, anxiety and discontent. It rewards dysfunction and wastes our wealth. Yet, no matter how many celebrities are touting it, or polar bears and third world islanders drowning from it, Americans aren't buying in to reducing GHG. That's why we're throwing in guaranteed fringe benefits like Losing Weight, Saving Money, Getting Fit, Better Sex, and many other Good Things.

The major sources of human generated GHG are described with affordable, practical solutions to really reduce them. We have a plan B to mitigate the predicted effects if we fail to make a dent in emitting GHG, and a plan C if the planet has already reached the tipping point. This guide includes individual baby step suggestions, larger social solutions and pipe dream possibilities. Even Al Gore could sell this package, but wait, wait- we're offering it to you for less than the cost of a feedlot fattened beef burger.

It's past time to really reduce GHG by changing the practices of the largest emitters. The mainstream media rarely identifies these sources because they are powerful and wealthy with sacred cow status. Raising concerns about GW without advocating effective actions, is just neurotic worry. Neurotic Worry only increases your risk of falling into the medical industrial system, a real energy/ money guzzler and very greenhouse gassy.

Chapter 1
A Heliocentric Solar System

The main Green House Gases (GHG) are Water Vapor, Carbon Dioxide, Methane, Nitrous Oxide and a few manufactured gases used for refrigeration. GHG absorb heat radiating outwards from our planet being cooked by the sun, otherwise we would broil by day and freeze by night. The percentage that human generated GHG contribute to warming compared to solar gain and other causes of GHG is a matter of debate, but the fact that they absorb heat and release it more slowly than other gases in the atmosphere is not.

Water vapor is rarely mentioned although it is is by far the largest proportion of GHG. That's why cloudy nights are warmer than clear ones, although clouds in the daytime reduce solar heating. Human activities like damming and irrigating increase water vapor, but oceanic evaporation and forest transpiration contributes most. Water vapor is essential, especially as precipitation, although rapid and sustained downpours can cause flooding. A predicted result of EWP.

Water Vapor provides 90% of the greenhouse effect in the atmosphere. The others have extremely different magnitudes of amounts, heating capacity and longevity in the atmosphere surrounding earth. Carbon Dioxide, CO_2 kicks in 90% of the remaining 10% of the Greenhouse effect. Methane is 30-40 times more heat absorbing than CO_2 over a century, while Nitrous Oxide, NO_2 is 300 times more potent. Luckily the other greenhouse gases are comparatively only a wisp of refrigerant leaks, because they range up to 1,500 times more potent than CO_2.

GHG absorb solar heat radiating away from the earth and act like a down blanket. This is not disputed and in general is a good thing for life on earth. The effect of human activity generating GHG on long range climate change is hotly disputed by pundits of all types. The majority of climatologists think human generated GHG are responsible for some, if not most of increasing global temperatures. An obstinate minority wants to wait and see.

It's also not disputed that levels of CO_2 in the atmosphere have nearly doubled since the dawn of the industrial age in the 17th century, from 200 parts per billion to 400. They have risen most rapidly in the last two hundred years, primarily from industrial societies burning fossil fuels. Carbon dioxide produced by burning fossil fuels is the major human source of GHG. Eighty five percent is from combusting Coal, Oil and Natural Gas for electricity generation, transportation and heating and cooling buildings.

Americans produce one fourth the GHG that humans of all nations emit, although China now produces more carbon dioxide than the U.S. They passed us in 2008 by burning coal to rapidly industrialize, but still only emit one fourth as much per person as Americans. European countries that are twice as efficient maintain a comfortable, industrial lifestyle, while most countries use less than one-fifth our rate. The third world aspires to AWOL so that could change. CO_2 is the GHG most industrial nations have signed treaties to reduce. The U.S. has declined so far, since China and other "developing" nations were given a pass. Even with carbon taxes, cap and trade and investing in "clean energy", most signatory countries didn't actually reduce emissions until the Great Recession. Germany did only by idling former East German power and manufacturing plants.

The amount of CO_2 humans generated increased dramatically when combustion machines began taking the place of human and animal power. Starting in England in the 1600's, the machine powered revolution spread across Europe then to America and around the globe, at least among the wealthier citizens. The Industrial Revolution was birthed by burning coal to fuel steam engines running pumps to drain water out of coal mines. Coal had been used to heat palaces and huts when wood and peat were scarce but combustion machines demanded regular feeding.

Steam engines were being used to pump, mill and locomote when the telegraph system synergistically boosted communication in the 19th. The second Industrial Revolution was calved in the twentieth century with coal fueled Electricity Generation lighting up buildings and running electric motors. Oil burning Internal Combustion engines won out for military vessels to replace mountains of coal at stations, then for motor vehicles and planes. Coal is still the main driver of human generation of CO_2 with China and India burning their vast seams of it to generate cheap electricity to jump start their entries in the next revolution.

Oceans and plants pull CO_2 out of the atmosphere and store it. What isn't captured lingers for decades in the atmosphere acting as a blanket for reflected solar heat. Human production of CO_2 climbed rapidly until 1927, when the Great Depression idled the Industrial Revolution for nearly a decade. Industrial manufacturing roared back with WWII, but had shifted to burning more oil, emitting considerably less GHG for the same energy output. Natural gas is cleaner burning than oil.

World production of CO_2 increased further when China, India, Brazil and other emerging economies joined in the industrial revolution. The global recession of 2008 dropped the levels produced 6% in one year, even for countries that hadn't signed the Kyoto Protocols. Global market collapse did more to reduce human GHG in one year than empty promises over a decade. Maybe the banksters deserved some cap and trade credits for crashing the global economy.

Global temperatures rose rapidly from the 1970's until the late 90's, then slowed in this century, due to decreased water vapor in the outer stratosphere according to the latest scientific finding. Lately they've said that the "slowing" was due to measurement error. Fear of GW because of GHG has been ramped up into media and cinematic hysteria but many Americans have tuned it out or don't believe the hype. Every storm, flood, tornado, drought or ice storm is blamed on GW, CC or EWP, while every record breaking cold spell is said to disprove GW depending on what side of the debate you're on.

The general thermometer trend has been hotter year round averages, even when punctuated by extremely long cold spells. Climate Change and Extreme Weather Phenomena became new terms entering the lexicon when the rise in recorded temperatures slowed somewhat, but this last decade was still the warmest one on record. Human recording of temperatures only goes back a century though.

A few meteorologists insist that blaming humans for GW is as geocentric as the Vatican was prior to Copernicus. They claim measurable changes in solar cycles are the main driver for heating up or cooling down the planet. They point out that several planets in the solar system are currently heating up, not just Earth. That the climate has changed considerably in the geological past, whether humans were around or not. Temperatures were this high 400-600 years ago before humans were emitting industrial levels of GHG.

The majority of political, scientific and media experts predict doom unless we cut back production and suck up existing GHG and stash them somewhere, Dissenters argue that the "near consensus" of scientists are rushing for the GW Express because 'There's gold in them thar hills'. Most Americans don't know who to believe about GW or what they can do to reduce GHG.

It's true that the Carbon Cap and Traders and the Nuclear Power Industry stand to gain hundreds of billions from current proposals to hitch their wagons to the GW Train. None of these will really reduce carbon dioxide. Both have posed as knights on white horses. Dissenters say they're two of the four horsemen of the Apocalypse.

The train boarders shout that solar radiation reaching our planet has diminished by 16% since 1985 and temperatures still climbed through the 90's. The platform sitters say temperatures have been dropping since 2002. The boarders say this was the hottest decade on record and the glaciers are melting like butter. The sitters find scientific errors and fraud when leading boarders fudge the numbers and hide evidence that doesn't support their claims. Those scandals damaged the climate change cause but fraud by GW opponents blow over heads stuck in denial sands.

Many skeptics are funded by fossil fuel conglomerates and business coalitions that have created 'front groups, fake citizens organizations and bogus scientific bodies" conspiring to spew doubt among voters, as a recent lawsuit by an Alaskan Inupiat tribe accused two dozen major fuel and utilities companies of doing.

Not all GW dissenters are in the pocket of the Coal, Oil, Cement, Automobile, Industrial and Nuclear Energy coalition, but even those not on COCAINE's payroll have been branded as bushwhackers by the GW crowd. The Bush Administration and Republicans gave deniers cover, while fighting a rearguard action against the media juggernaut of environmental doomsayers. The Obama administration passed higher fuel efficiency standards down the road, but they're doing little to reduce them now. His Secretary of State, John Kerry recently mocked climate change "deniers", calling their science "shoddy" to an Indonesian audience. "Nor should we allow any room for those who think the costs associated with doing the right thing outweigh the benefits."

The mainstream media is firmly in the GW camp, except for Fox News talking heads. That station has used dissenting weathermen to deny the consensus. They are singing to their choir, just as the mainstream is yodeling to theirs. Most Americans have tuned it out. The anti- PR campaign denying GW is funded by industries that emit the most GHG, and has persuaded over half of Americans to their viewpoint, although most citizens aren't that concerned, because it feels out of their control.

Chapter 2
Time for New Slogans

I first wrote about GHG and GW in 1979 when Jimmy Carter was president and I was a student at the University of Florida. In an opinion piece for the UF Gator, I called for transforming transportation by supporting cycling, walking and mass transit to reduce pollution from motor vehicles, listing reducing greenhouse gases to prevent global warming as one reason. My source was Howard Odum, a UF professor who birthed the field of systems biology.

I love to say I told you so, but my journalistic jeremiads were never influential and virtually forgotten, unless I bring it up. If we'd followed Jimmy Carter's advice and worn sweaters and put solar panels on our roofs, we might not have gotten to this state of imminent catastrophe. Then again that's part of why he wasn't re-elected.

The corporate megaphones we have for a free press have been baying about GW at least since Bill Clinton's presidency. These have increased to dire warning hysteria in the last decade since Hurricane Katrina. That's as good a reason as any to doubt the hype, because when the corporate media focuses on an environmental issue, it's always around generating future profits for their owners and advertisers.

The last time they were bleating this loudly about an environmental issue was around Acid Rain. All claimed success when the feds passed Acid Rain cap and trade legislation to reduce U.S. production of sulfates and other causes of Acid Rain. This was accomplished almost entirely by shipping manufacturing off to third world countries without annoying environmental regulations around sulfur emissions. Now the experts are saying that Acid Rain protected against GW because sulfate particles in clouds reflect more sunlight back into space. Luckily, China is taking up our slack in spewing sulfites, along with surging into the lead in GHG production.

Most countries that signed the Kyoto Treaty did not reduce their GHG to 1990 levels. Only West Germany did it by uniting with East Germany and shutting down their aging, coal powered industrial factories. If the U.S. had ratified Kyoto and other international treaties in Bali or Copenhagen, it's unlikely we'd have achieved GHG reductions either. The political will for the systemic changes required is lacking.

Political will comes from changing beliefs and behaviors. As individuals we can make and promote affordable, lifestyle changes. We can organize with other people who also feel helpless and hopeless as lone individuals to drive changes. We are the vanguard called on to help an industrial society evolve into a sustainable one.

Unless China, India, Brazil and other third word emerging economies are included in any global treaty, human generated GHG will increase because they are rapidly industrializing with the dirtiest fuel source, coal. Some economists predict we can only slow the growth of fossil fueled emissions at enormous cost. Protecting against predicted damage can be funded by going full steam ahead to keep the economy roaring.

Emerging economies want to climb into western civilization with AWOL as the pinnacle. The U.S. claims it refuses to sign on because China won't, and they won't because we won't. It's a Catch 22. The full court press about GW overwhelmed our short attention span, and we are suffering from disaster exhaustion. Who can keep it all straight?

Americans definitely don't want higher fuel prices. Oil companies are ripping us off already. It's just easier to ignore a slow moving catastrophe, especially if there's nothing we can do to avoid it. If only saving the planet fit in with our more pressing concerns. That's why it's time for a new slogan, a better way forward that does all good things for everyone, except those GHG emitters who refuse to evolve. Americans are ready for class warfare, eager to punish those greedy bastards who got us into this financial depression. This plan will accomplish that too.

Chapter 3
Addiction Creates Necessity

Many environmentalists think GW hysteria is the only way to scare people into cutting back on energy consumption. Doomsday scenarios are unlikely to accomplish this goal, whether accurate about future weather or not. GW hysteria will not be effective at persuading most Americans to reduce GHG because we are addicted to generating them. Addictions aren't behaviors persuasive to reason or influenced by future negatives.

Obama has talked about GHG reductions and passed future fuel efficiency regulations, but a divided congress will not take effective actions unless we the people lead. We need to know where we want to get to and how to do it, or leading is futile.

Are human generated GHG the major cause of GW or just a fart in the wind? Are the dire predictions for Climate Change merely substituting a scientific environmental doomsday for a religious apocalyptic tale? Clarifying this debate is beyond most Americans understanding of climate science, mine included, so that is not my mission. Evangelizing for adopting a greener economy/lifestyle to Lose Weight, Save Money and Really Reduce GHG is.

This book aims to illuminate the major sources of GHG, propose affordable solutions to lower them and point out the many personal benefits gained by doing so. Whether we can change the climate by reducing our carbon footprint is debatable. But the facts are undisputed that we can become healthier and save tons of money by massively reducing our energy consumption. Those are far more compelling reasons for Americans than avoiding another predicted doomsday or saving a few polar bears.

Most of our GHG production is associated with spewing Toxic Waste of one kind or another into the environment, which includes our bodies, babies and pets. GHG emissions also cause the production of a wide variety substances known to harm the ecology, human health and the general welfare. Despite the PR Hype, Toxic Waste is not good for us. Lower GHG means less Toxic Waste.

Neither Americans nor the citizens of industrializing nations will cut back on a fossil fuel guzzling lifestyle or aspirations for having one based on guilt or fear alone. Bureaucratic regulations, financial penalties and even stronger methods will have to be applied to torque us into compliance. If the doomsday predictions for Climate Change are true, then the puny measures that experts and policy wonks are proposing to reduce GHG to Slow GW now, will prove as futile as organizing a bailing brigade on the Titanic.

Maybe, if we'd listened to President Jimmy Carter in the 70's, instead of making fun of his gay sweater. If we'd made conservation a cornerstone of a rational energy policy then, we could've saved our coasts from the predicted flooding and super storms, and the heartland from sizzling droughts and killer tornados. We didn't and the pace of preparation is too little, too late. It's past time to start preparing for the hazards our society is predicted to face from floods, fires, storms, heat waves and droughts. These will be accompanied with escalating energy costs that will cripple AWOL more than terrorist Muslims ever have.

The "solutions" being pushed by experts and policy wonks are little more than cynical and self serving snake oil to further enrich and empower the governing agencies and corporations pushing for them. They position the people to plunge into the deluge because they ignore the biggest elephants.

Yes, Virginia there are highly effective actions we can take as individuals, citizens, organizations and governing bodies that will Save Money, Lower Energy Bills, Reduce Greenhouse Gases, Toxic Waste and Acid Rain. All while Feeling Better, Losing Weight with whiter teeth. Guaranteed.

Chapter 4
The Cult of the Military

America's military is the single largest consumer of oil in the world. Even after reducing their energy use by 60% over the last twenty years by closing bases they are the world's largest user of energy. They've built up a ginormous carbon footprint since WWII making the world safe for democracies when they do what they're told, military juntas when not. Since these gases can last a century in the upper atmosphere, the DOD would have to plant an original Amazonian forest of trees to become carbon neutral for all their past sins. They don't seem especially concerned about preventing GW by lowering their carbon footprint, even though they've named it the number one security threat of the 21st century.

Most of their energy reduction came from closing bases after the Cold War ended. Even in the flush of victory it was like pulling teeth to actually reduce the rate of increase in the military budget. Shedding bases with their energy sucking buildings and facilities allowed them to reduce their electricity usage to only 10% of their total energy consumption. Now 75% of their energy use is oil, mostly for materials and supplies transported in myriad planes, trucks and ships.

Yet all the conservation and efficiency regulations passed by the military have been aimed at buildings and facilities, not their vehicles. There are no gas "sipping" tanker jets, no hybrid aircraft carriers or tanks.   No federal legislation aimed at reducing GHG targets the military budget or even its fuel efficiency. Since Defense costs more than half of their discretionary spending, this should be a no-brainer.

Half the oil burnt goes to the Air Force, mostly as jet fuel, of which 85% is used to move more fuel to the battlefield. These figures are from Sohbet Karbuz of Energy Times, who cautions that they are based on DOD disclosures and don't include unpaid oil and outsourcing of military activities, so actual amounts are higher. He points out that the quantities used by the military are so enormous they are calculated at gallons per mile and barrels per hour. Each American soldier fighting in Iraq and Afghanistan to protect our freedoms at home were using 16 gallons of oil per day. In 2001, the Defense Science Board found that "the fully burdened costs of [military] fuel", the commodity price plus delivery and treatment for casualties from driving fuel tankers in Iraq, was "at least $20 a gallon and for many missions went upwards of hundreds of dollars per gallon for ground forces." Airborne delivery cost $42 a gallon.

The fully burdened costs of gasoline for American consumers include military protection of oil supplies and routes, subsidies and tax breaks for oil companies, road building, widening and repairing, stormwater damage expenses, traffic enforcement, medical treatment for collisions and environmental pollution. Estimates range from $15-25 a gallon of subsidized costs. Neither drivers nor the military pay full costs for fuel, passing most off to future generations.

In *Hot, Flat and Crowded*, Thomas Friedman quotes a DOD analyst, "in just one small forward operating base we were bringing in 10,000 gallons a day of diesel," using 9,000 gallons of it in electrical generators. Ninety five per cent of the power was used to air condition tents in120 degree heat. That's why 70% of the U.S. Central Command's energy budget went to move fuel from one base to another.

After 5 years of pouring diesel into these tent holes, they began to insulate them with commercially available foam achieving 40-75% reductions in air conditioning costs. Then they erected large domes with foamed exteriors and a more blast resistant concrete inner layer powered by wind turbines and solar panels. They're probably green mosques now that we've fled that Pottery Barn, but affordable green housing for Americans is no longer available even in Iraqi military zones.

The DOD reduced their energy use significantly since 1985 by shuttering bases and downsizing troops. The War on Terror considerably boosted their GHG emissions since 9/11. Our military expanded into the policeman for the planet while supporting corporate profits, imperial aims and the comfort and joy of our citizens.

After President Carter's conservation pleas were hooted down in 1979, he issued the Carter Doctrine in January 1980 at the direction of the Council of Foreign Relations and the Trilateral Commission. This Doctrine announced a more muscular Jimmy with lust for oil in his heart. It stated that the secure flow of oil in the Middle East was "in the vital interests of the United States of America" and "any means necessary, even military" would be used to protect this. This was as significant as the Monroe Doctrine, which claimed all of South America to be in our sphere of influence.

Michael Klare, professor of Peace and Energy Security of Hampshire College reports the U.S. military has essentially become a Global Oil Protection Service since then. Vast lakes of oils are burned defending overseas sources and shipped oil and natural gas, patrolling pipelines and sea routes for America and its allies.

One hundred billion dollars, one-fourth of the DOD's budget, not including the War on Iraq and Afghanistan goes to Persian Gulf protection and patrolling. The Carter Doctrine has multiplied like a hydra headed monster protecting oil supplies in the Caspian Sea, Columbia, Nigeria and beyond.

The U.S. uses 1/4 the petroleum on the planet, so it's understandable we want to protect and maybe even seize oil supplies. It's natural when you're as addicted as we are to oil to be spending more and more time and money securing a steady supply. Our military/industrial complex as Eisenhower warned is a leviathan sucking up oil and gushing greenhouse gases. Yet "GW experts" or well meaning legislators rarely mention this steaming dragon as the obvious place to cut out GHG.

Military contracts are ladled out in every congressional district, to the medical/academic complex, industrial suppliers and service outsourcing companies. Even after closing hundreds of bases, thousands more are scattered around the country and planet. Defense Department outsourcing is all the rage, each contractor needing their own buildings, fleets and warehouses. Defending our addiction to oil sucks up energy, money with a flume of Toxic Waste and GHG.

It's a tragedy that the idea of Humanity coming together to Create Peace seems Delusional. Ever since the first tribe decided it was easier to take than to make or trade goods, war has attained a certain historical imperative. It's our fixed belief in the Cult of the Military that makes even our gargantuan military seem sane to the majority of citizens, as long as we can afford our next fix of oil based energy. This transfers into the militarization of police forces primarily driven by the forty year War on Drugs, mainly marijuana. Shifting that belief in society will be more revolutionary and GHG reducing than changing out a few million light bulbs. It will save trillions, too.

National Security, Department of Defense and their myriad contractors are funded like pashas, not just to protect our automobile addicted, air conditioned, suburban sprawled lifestyle, though. The military must have oil to fuel their imperial activity. This is why it is defined as a vital, national interest. When a shortage of petroleum becomes severe or is contrived to be, the military will get the lion's share. We'll be rationed like in WWII, although probably by price. What's left over will go to government duties, emergency response and policing the gas riots.

Soldiers who were fighting in hellish conditions in Iraq to keep oil flowing at home probably built up some resentment after being sent repeatedly to sacrifice so much, while lazy citizens were leaving the petroleum tap open on the home front. They noticed that opposition to the War in Iraq didn't even register until gasoline went up to $3 a gallon. When the military is ordered to help restore order in the streets over fuel shortage riots, they might just lob in some cluster bombs.

As GHG pacifists, we have to think strategically and act tactically to slice through the claims and propaganda of the military industrial complex. Pacifists have other strengths though. Our minds are more attuned to cooperation across tribal, ethnic, linguistic trenches. We can act en masse yet autonomously, self guided in parallel processes, to find the chinks in the armor of the behemoth.

As citizens we can vote, even campaign for candidates who have vowed to limit our military spending to defending our national borders. Such candidates are already on many ballots. To Really Reduce GHG Americans can simply vote for someone they've never heard of. Curing political apathy is more difficult than losing weight. Adopt simple voting strategies to achieve progressive goals. You won't find many "serious" candidates with Dismantle the Military/Industrial

Complex.on their platform. Candidates who are ignored or ridiculed by the corporate media are those who took no corporate money to buy ads.

Voting by itself won't make much difference, but it's an easy and revolutionary act. When Hope and Change they can believe in lures youth into the booths, their hopes are dashed. Many vote against their own self and class interests, swayed by biased media and ads. Once we begin to define our national and international interests by what makes us healthy, relatively happy and sufficiently safe, we will be well on our way to Saving the Planet. Kumbay Yah, and all.

Taking even 10% from the military budget to fund General Welfare and Domestic Tranquility at home would stimulate our economy and create more jobs than spending it on Imperial Overreach. Back away from militarization abroad and reject the complete militarization of the Home Land. The Wars on Drugs targets mainly minorities and poor, imprisons more citizens than any other country, failed to reduce drug use or rehabilitate prisoners and costs far more than social supports that have been proven to reduce crime, addiction, poor health, teenage pregnancy, school dropout and unemployment rates. This would empty out the concrete and steel prison industrial complexes, sucking up energy and spewing out GHG to provide jobs for rural economies. Replace those jobs and secured prison cells with healthier, reform work on organic farms providing real rehabilitation

The military mindset is firmly embedded in the national psyche. Armed forces and their vast network of suppliers and procurers seem like an unstoppable juggernaut. This is a huge task, which even true believers despair over achieving. That's no reason to give up hope and get all despondent, just develop a long term strategy. We're on a long count calendar of evolution. If the last Prince of Peace got crucified for trying to erode the war machine, our road is infinitely easier. We'll have to get down in the trenches and put our shoulders to the wagon, when the star we hitched it to get bogged down in the quagmire.

Chapter 5
Electric Avenue

Generating Electricity or is usually named as the largest source of GHG in the US, because the military is the elephant in the tent that no one mentions. Most of their GHG are generated outside the country anyways. Electricity generation is primarily used to make government, commercial and residential edifices habitable.

Transportation to move between buildings has also been fingered as the leading source of GHG depending on who is estimating. Numbers vary, but making cement for buildings and infrastructure using natural gas is the third largest source of GHG. although industrial manufacturing is also listed as the third major source of CO_2 at 24-28% of the total. Dow Chemical saved 8 billion dollars from 1995 to 2009 by reducing energy use.

Photovoltaic solar panels on every roof won't magically make the American Way of Life (AWOL) sustainable. That will take another Great Awakening as transformative as the first three Industrial Revolutions. The first was kicked into gear by steam engines, the second by electrical and internal combustion engines and the third with computerized communication, all building on the creative destruction of the last one.

Power plants that generate electricity waste up to 60% as heat. In Scandinavia, they've built co-generation plants that heat other buildings nearby with the exhaust. Two thirds of the electricity generated is lost conducting it through vast grids of power lines delivering it to widely distributed users. That heat could be captured by more than birds' toes. Instead of burying or stringing power lines around cities and towns, encasing them in thick rubber pedestrian paths and bike lanes would melt winter snow and ice, creating year round paths without plows.

Government and commercial buildings use huge baseloads of electricity. They can conserve more energy than photovoltaic can generate at one third the cost. Wal-Mart reduced energy use by 45% in their pilot green SuperStore using evaporative cooling, radiant heating, natural light and more efficient refrigeration. Oak Ridge National Laboratory says that by retrofits and smart designs 200 million tons of carbon could be saved a year. Commercial building owners have little incentive to retrofit however, since their tenants pay the utilities.

Around 40% of residential energy use is for heating water or air. Solar thermal is three times more efficient than solar electric for these functions. . Using roofs and walls with southern exposure for thermal solar water and heat storage, clothes dryers, ovens and incinerating toilets is far more cost effective than solar panels generating electricity to run inefficient appliances. Photovoltaic is most efficient at charging storage batteries for direct current (DC) light, electronics and electric motors.

Public, commercial and residential electricity use could be halved with current technology and retrofitting. Since public and commercial buildings use 36%, while residential is anywhere from 20-36%, that's dozens of new coal fired power plants not needed. If the military wasn't hoovering $80 billion a year in research and development monies for "defense", we could easily triple the efficiency of buildings.

Economic theory claims decisions by most individuals and companies to invest in retrofitting to reduce GHG will be based on cost/savings, not whether the source is carbon neutral. The carbon cap and trade market, (already up and running in Europe and California) charges fees based on carbon dioxide emitted to pay for measures to reduce them. With trillions of potential trading units at play financial institutions are eager to trade. Most Americans will have to pay more for electricity and fuel to fund this financial carousel. More will blame the polar bear than the carbon traders.

Coal is the cheapest fuel for power plants, but the fracking bonanza lowered the price of natural gas and oil to near parity. The main benefit from fracking is killing off financial market interest in building new nuclear or coal powered plants. Coal will be hit hardest by any carbon tax, because it is the dirtiest. Burning coal can be far cleaner with existing technology but electricity producers have successfully resisting retrofitting their aging plants. Forcing existing plants to upgrade will save people's health and the environment while working to phase them out.

The west coast is breathing toxic dust from China's coal fired plants. The east coast is showered with mercury from plants in the Midwest. With carbon taxes, coal fired power plants will cost more to run. King Coal has plans to sequester carbon dioxide underground in the mines they abandoned when they began scraping mountains into molehills. That would be good for our health, but raise electric bills. When the price of electricity and gasoline increase with carbon trading markets, most Americans will use less. The wealthiest will not be seriously affected and they can profit from investments in this new market.

Homeowners cut back on energy efficiency projects in the recession because they couldn't afford the upfront costs, although savings can pay back in several years. One survey found that only a quarter would do so even if they had an extra ten grand to put into their castles. The rest would invest in granite countertops to flip their crib.

The price per kilowatt of photovoltaic solar panels used to only make economic sense for buildings off the power line grid by a mile or more, or to power DC lights and electronics. They're so much cheaper now that their costs pencil out, although their efficiency is still low. Solyndra promised to double efficiency from dawn to dusk, but was undone by cheap, inefficient panels flooding in from China. Their government made massive investments in manufacturing them to enter the 21st century while our government basically abandoned renewable energy. Making solar power the poster child of reducing GHG is basically greenwash, because China is using coal fired power plants to manufacture them. Putting photovoltaic solar panels on every roof won't change that.

If we can't massively reduce our use of electricity, we'll be force-fed "clean" nuclear power and "cleaner" coal to generate our demand. Aging nuclear power stations are routinely being given 20 year extensions by the NEC to generate 20 per cent more electricity than they were cranking out for thirty years. These 20/200 approvals are blind faith, considering alarming safety and maintenance records. Tons of spent radioactive are fuel fuming away in holding ponds waiting for a final resting place. It's no surprise that nuclear power has jumped on the GHG bandwagon, although electricity from nukes generates almost as much GHG as natural gas. More if counting total fuel cycle from mining to storage in a secure site for the next quarter million years. They release huge amounts of heated water that kill fish while their holding ponds are a tempting terrorist target.

They can't be built without huge government subsidies and guarantees, so of course our politicians chip in. Obama's energy policy includes almost $90 billion in subsidies for new nukes. Still better than Bush's which plotted a preemptive war on Iraq to secure its oil fields. There's far cheaper and cleaner ways to boil water for steam turbines than radioactive uranium. Parabolic mirrors could accomplish the same result using solar power.

Clean coal is a joke, as funny as ethanol from corn for fuel. Yes, the feds are quite humorous when it comes to solving our energy crisis. Unfortunately, their lame solutions will become our grim future if we don't focus on reducing electricity and fuel use besides generating more 'renewable' energy. Despite the most upbeat predictions of renewable resources, the most immediate and cheapest energy source is massive conservation through individual, social and structural changes.

Other pie in the sky solutions like hydrogen power and fusion will waste time and money better spent on conserving energy. We can improve and install appropriate wind, hydro, solar, bio-fuel technologies, but depending on Washington hype to promote alternatives is futile, when their giveaways to coal, oil, corn and nuclear are so massive. That will remain the case as long as federal campaigns remain funded by special interest money.

Chapter 6
Sustainable Castles

When it comes to Reducing Greenhouse Gases, Saving Money and Losing Weight, nothing is more pivotal than AWOL. Symbolized by our starter castles secluded in the suburbs and exurbs from crowded cities, tied in by the grid of highways, powerlines, coaxial cables, water and sewage pipes, stuffed to the brim with plugged in modern conveniences and electronic devices, sucking energy from their three car garages to their under insulated attics. These piles consume enormous amounts of energy to supply their water and sewer, provide their heating and cooling, run their major and minor appliances, fuel their oversized vehicles parked beside the green, grass lawn.

There's skyscraper office towers with plate glass windows and underground vaults, cavernous malls, supermarkets and Big Box stores with their feeder supply warehouses. There are storage units for the stuff we can't fit, restaurant rows and retail strips.

The shelters we build for residence, employment, recreation, consuming, manufacturing and imprisonment emit 38% of GHG in America. Every phase of their existence is carbon intensive from steel and concrete foundations to trucking away deconstruction rubble. The construction trade is hugely greenhouse gassy. The edifices built and maintained are enormously wasteful in design and location. If we're serious about cutting enough GHG to make a dent in GW then our buildings must fundamentally change. Tweaking their design a little to get a gold star for "green" construction is a false start.

Generating electricity to run buildings is the second largest source of GHG in the U.S. Forty one percent of average home energy use is electrical, while twice that is lost in the transmission from power plants. Without electricity delivered through relatively fragile infrastructure, most buildings are as helpless as baby seals. Another forty per cent of residential energy use was natural gas, 11% petroleum and 4% renewable in 2009. Heating blows through half of home energy costs, with cooling using a tenth, depending on geography. In residential houses, major appliances use half the electricity, water heaters account for 12% of energy use, and electronics cost 8-20% of electric bills.

Making cement to construct buildings by burning limestone at 1600 degrees Fahrenheit is the third largest source of GHG. Manufacturing plate glass windows, steel beams and doors produces huge amounts of GHG. Wood for lumber fells trees that might live for centuries storing carbon, to be used briefly for framing concrete or in structures that may not last decades.

There are far more sustainable building materials and designs using less embedded energy that keep buildings cooler in the heat and warmer in the cold. These range from adobe or cob, mud brick or rammed earth tubes, straw bales or clay slip, bamboo, canvas or felt. Aerated concrete is a fire proof, sound proof, light brick that actually absorbs CO2 and stores it for centuries. Some of these materials are cheaper than conventional building materials, are fire proof, inhibit mold and improve indoor air, but require more hands on labor to build them. Higher labor costs make them prohibitive in our value system, even though they are far more affordable to heat, cool and maintain over their lifetime, and those jobs are better, greener and can't be outsourced.

Most of what's called sustainable or green now is usually only a little less unsustainable. Dwell magazine showcases how the wealthy typically squander even more resources when they go green and "sustainable". Much of the green marketplace is only selling virtuous luxury. Recently, in Marin County, California a couple whose tech company went public wanted to build their dream green castle. So they tore down the $20 million dollar palace they bought for its location to go green.

We can't all live in mansions. "sustainable" or not. The average new house has ballooned from 1000 square feet in the 50's when they had much larger families, to around 2,700 today. In some zip codes 4,000 sq. ft. is a tear down. New homes are forty five percent larger since 1970. New construction was mostly on hold during the Great Recession except for luxury homes, but building new "green" palaces to replace a multi-million dollar teardown will not change the majority of our built environment.

As utilitarian spaces, not many houses are actually worth what they are valued at. American style houses are beasts to maintain. If you're not cleaning something, you're fixing something. If you can't do it yourself, you're at the mercy of the home repair gauntlet. That doesn't even include permitting fees and contractor headaches.

Transportation was the major energy consumer then before fuel efficiency standards, while ballooning buildings are now the major source of emissions after electrical generation from coal plants. Buildings and their occupants consume much of the electricity, although more transportation is electric now.

The 2003 book, *Cradle to Cradle* by Michael Braungart and William McDonough was influential in the sustainable design world. The authors worked with Ford motor company to build a massive automobile assembly plant River Rouge, MI. Its living roof lowered stormwater abatement costs by millions. They worked with Brad Pitt to build affordable, non-toxic houses for Hurricane Katrina victims in New Orleans.

They helped NASA build the greenest research center in Silicon Valley, the 50,000 sq .ft Sustainability Base. It came in on budget, and uses magnitudes less water and energy than most office buildings. Oddly enough, they were asked to work with NASA to design something to survive on Mars, but convinced the space agency to build for thriving on Earth instead.

There are three times as many houses as there are family units in the untied states. Some are foreclosed, maybe uninhabitable, but most are second or third houses squandering almost as much energy and resources empty, as with a houseless family moved in. We don't need to build new affordable housing or homeless shelters. Simply repeal the tax code that gives write offs for second homes, or at least third ones. John McCain couldn't even remember how many he owned during his losing 2008 campaign.

There will be significantly more empty office, manufacturing and shopping spaces if the Main Street economy can't struggle out of the ravine Wall Street drove it into. The mall parking lots will be barren if this recession regroups, unless they're parking FEMA trailers and RV's for the mortgage broken.

The single largest purchase and investment for most Americans is their home, yet banks charge four times the sticker price with interest over 30 years. When you consider how carbon intensive every aspect of our economy is, that extra expense compounds our carbon. Hundreds of thousands of Americans had to walk away from "underwater" houses, owing the banks more than they're worth. This was long before predicted rising oceans from GW. Others were forced to leave ancestral manses they used as piggy banks to borrow money on.

Retrofitting existing houses and buildings to make them more efficient, healthier and cheaper to maintain would provide more value to the occupants and generate millions of jobs. Using existing technology and practices, the U.S. could cut 1.3 billion tons of CO_2 according to the Oak Ridge National Laboratory. These will pay for themselves in savings over their lifetime. Zero percent interest loans to property owners to invest in efficiency would stimulate the economy, save money and really reduce GHG. The biggest banks have been given those terms since their bailout to stimulate the economy, although they've hoarded more than they loaned for creating jobs. Most was used to buy other banks or stashed in interest bearing bonds to use for the next crisis.

It's not just how structures are built, but where. Suburbs and Exurbs sprawled across former farmland from sea to shining sea emit half the GHG of all residential buildings, even though far more people live in urban complexes and high rises. The carbon footprint of these suburban and rural estates could be narrowed by building green second and third units for young farmers on the property. Affordable housing can be the green shack out back. A 200 sq ft residence is plenty big enough for a tidy couple with no baggage.

Their small home catches rain off the roof to store several thousand gallons in inflatable tubes insulating the north side. Photovoltaic and solar thermal provide electricity, charge batteries and provide heating needs. The south facing attached greenhouse purifies their used waters with Living

Systems ponds that feed fish and provide irrigation to their extensive garden. The primary homeowner gains income or assistance, while providing affordable housing and suburban infill. The lawn becomes organic garden and fruit orchard, their help is on site living in a post disaster resource center from the coming SuperStorms.

These can even be built without building permits in the international "green" building code adopted in CA, and being adopted around the untied states. Suburbs, icons of AWOL can be transformed by building what people need. Suburbs were glorified as the epitome of American Freedom after WWII, returning veterans supported in buying a detached home with a spot of green lawn and raising a brood, when a working dad could support a stay at home mom.

The fenced in yard, meant privacy to retreat indoors to an air conditioned nightmare as Henry Miller dubbed it. Suburban sprawl intertwined with millions of miles of asphalt because motor vehicles are essential to these separated silos. Residents in some dense urban areas or small town pockets may not need to own automobiles for basic mobility, but even these few pedestrian/cyclist/transit enabled oases are supported logistically by truck and car traffic. Every community is riven with the danger, noise, air and water pollution of motor vehicles.

Construction and Transportation contributions to GHG are co-mingled in America. Motor vehicle transportation is required to build, maintain, supply and get to and away from our buildings and uses 34% of energy in America. Transportation generates 60% of GHG in California, mainly because of wider sprawl and milder winter weather, but also because buildings are far more efficient here than most of the untied states.

Right now, the wealthiest Americans get richer and thinner, while the rest struggle to keep a roof overhead. The average American house consumes more energy than a Chinese sweatshop and puts out more waste. Residential solar power is perfect for running efficient lights and electronics and charging batteries for electric motors. Photovoltaic panels make great shade structures over parking lots, reducing GW from heat buildup of the black asphalt and metal cars. Painting roads, parking lots and roofs white, would cause a similar reduction in urban heat islands.

Advances in solar power, both thermal and electric, have made it possible for homes to be self sufficient in energy, and sell some back to the grid during peak hours. Windmills have gotten smaller and quieter for distributed residential use, while they've grown enormously for industrial generation. There are known hazards and environmental problems from wind generation, although certainly far less than nuclear and coal fired plants. However, comparing them to the worst to defend their unmitigated placement and design is not likely to solve those issues.

The water wasted in American houses and offices creates significant GHG just by piping it in as purified and out as sewage. The largest single user of electricity in California are the water pumps bringing Bay Area delta water over the Tehachapi mountains to Los Angeles. The largest electricity user in Marin county, California is the Marin Municipal Water District. Agriculture uses 80% of water in California, but domestic use still sucks on an enormous straw.

Amazingly, most water isn't used for drinking, cooking, bathing, or even swimming pools and hot tubs. Landscape irrigation is the end use of most residential potable water, mostly for lawns. Push lawnmowers put out more pollution than 11 cars, riding mowers equal 344 cars. The ongoing drought in California has created a groundswell against grass, although there are varieties that are drought tolerant.

An organic garden and orchard could be grown with graywater, stored raincatch or biologically purified sewage. Instead we mix gray water from showers with toilet and kitchen sink blackwater and flush it away to a buried septic or distant sewage system. This complex requires more energy to purify it enough to dump it into the nearest body of water. It may be "pure" but it is still toxic to marine life.

Even "non-failing" permitted septic systems are polluting groundwater, creeks, springs and surrounding seas, while exacerbating the drainage problems where clustered. The migration of pathogens in groundwater is implicit in regulations allowing certain levels of nitrate along with other unregulated pollutants including phosphates, heavy metals, pesticides, petrochemical, chemical and pharmaceutical byproducts, caffeine and other drugs, radioactive elements, bacteria and viruses. These are known groundwater contaminants from septic systems, with increased levels from failing and unregulated systems.

They migrate into drinking water, both into source supplies and through the semi-permeable nature of buried water pipes. Larger scale sewage systems are just as polluting when they function as designed. Large rainstorms typically dump more water into the drainage system than they are engineered to handle with millions of gallons of untreated sewage spills from storm surges, clogs or breaks in aging, stressed sewer pipes.

The engineered running water system we take for granted is integral to AWOL. It relies on vast dammed reservoirs filling up with silt, miles of subterranean pipes built in the last century and frequently crumbling. They link treatment plants to sanitize water for drinking with homes and commercial buildings that then commingle water used for almost everything but drinking into sewage pipes flowing to massive treatment plants that filter and sterilize it enough to dump in the nearest body of water. The expense of maintaining water and sewage infrastructure is growing for cities and taxpayers, breaking the budgets of some. It has a huge carbon footprint and is unsustainable where climate change brings extended drought.

We squander water because we can. It's relatively cheap, but no matter how many low flush toilets are installed, flushing away crap is a total waste. It could be composted along with food waste, yard clippings, and biodegradable plastic. Compost cooks with microbial action up to 160 degrees, killing pathogens and creating fertilizer. Sewage waste can be purified using microbial and plant processes in closed greenhouses.

Sim Van der Ryn proposed using a solar aquaculture sewage system in his 1986 design for a Solar Village at Hamilton Air Force Base in Marin County after the military shuttered it. His proposed model was Solar Aquasystems of San Diego's innovative wastewater treatment design using microorganisms in greenhouse heated ponds. Van der Ryn was California's state architect when Governor Jerry Brown was still known as "Moonbeam" for his crazy ideas about energy and water conservation, bicycle transportation, rock star girlfriends and Zen meditation. Thirty years later the new, serious, married Governor Jerry Brown is officially concerned about GW, of course, but he's for fracking and intent on high speed rail and water tunnel boondoggles.

Van der Ryn launched a massive state building program in the 70's that focused on energy efficiency, use of solar and renewable resources. His design for the Solar Village in Marin would have been affordable to build and to live in, with the design emphasis on creating a walkable community. Novato authorities chose a conventional design instead.

John Todd, director of The New Alchemy Institute in Cape Cod, Massachusetts used the principles of ecology or bio-mimicry to design bio shelters in the 70's. These free standing Plexiglas domes or attached greenhouses can purify sewage or graywater using biological processes. Omega Institute in Rhinebeck, New York built a Living System based on these principles to process sewage from their three season workshops and retreats. This had been treated in their septic system causing extensive algae and plant blooms in Long Pond, the lake they front on.

These living systems can be added to single family residences or multi-family complexes to purify both their flush toilet sewage and shower and sink graywater. The bio-shelters generate nutrients that feed fish and nourish garden soils. They use half the energy of industrial fish farming to gain ten times the productivity. The water flows out pure enough to irrigate crops and trees with.

Rain catch and Graywater can irrigate gardens and orchards or even be biologically filtered to re-use as potable water. The lawns Americans endlessly water, fertilize, pesticide and mow could be productive Victory Gardens, if we got patriotic about the War on GW. Americans typically view conserving energy like Ronald Reagan did, as "being cold in the winter and hot in the summer". That kind of hair shirting will never be popular, while wasting energy is seen as total luxury. The journey to become more sustainable needs to show Americans that conservation is cheaper, healthier, sexier and easy.

Going beyond the U.S. Green Building Council's Leadership in Energy and Environmental Design (LEED) certified construction to compete in the Living Building Challenge (LBC) will be the new frontier in reducing the GHG production from new and renovated homes and commercial buildings. Its creator, James McLennan, compares these buildings to flowers, both rooted in place, able to extract all the energy and water they need from their surroundings, providing habitat while being beautiful and non-polluting.

He developed seven petals, or performance areas that buildings are judged on with 23 imperatives contained in their parameters. Limits to Growth demands using already developed sites or renovate existing structures. The Car Free Living imperative encourages denser mixed neighborhoods with areas set aside for food production.

They must be energy net producers using renewable, onsite sources to meet the Energy Petal's Net Zero Energy imperative. This is the petal that most green building has focused on, with numerous competitions like the U.S. Department of Energy's Solar Decathlon- nine day competitions that college teams have competed in since 2005. Winning teams have designed affordable, practical homes of 600-1000 sq. ft that supply all their own energy and maintain comfortable indoor environments over 24 hours.

The Water petal of LBC aims to create water independent buildings and neighborhoods, relying on rain catch storage and/or wells without chemical treatment, using only UV sterilization and physical or biological filters. When conflicting with outdated code requirements, builders must appeal to appropriate agencies to remove these barriers to self sufficiency.

The Health petal pushes the envelope for developers to create cleaner indoor air, natural light, and consider their structure's relation to its environment, seeking to integrate it into the environment in a biophilic imperative.

The Materials petal measures the embodied energy, toxic chemicals, fair labor and sustainable extraction of materials, and pressuring manufacturers to redesign their product if no acceptable materials are available. Upcycle employs similar standards for non-toxic materials and has changed the industry by asking it to focus on safety and health.

Petals that set this standard apart from most "green" building designs are the Social Equity and Beauty petals. They emphasize internal access for disabled and the community to external infrastructure and natural waterways, sunlight and fresh air imperatives for quality of life.

Retrofitting existing buildings to reduce their energy and money sucking habits is essential for Americans to really reduce GHG. Simply weather fitting with available products alone would conserve more energy than extracting toxic Canadian Tar Sands. Choosing to exploit every last reservoir of petroleum instead of conservation will generate enough GHG to mean game over for GW. Inertia and unwillingness to spend capital on conservation are obstacles as large as fossil fuel opposition.

Emphasize that this investment in America will reduce the financial stress of staying sheltered or making and selling products. Retrofitting can be done for half the cost of our failed adventure in Iraq. Millions of high paying jobs will be created that can't be exported. Billions will be saved on energy costs and massive amounts of GHG will not be released. Lose Weight and Save Money, win/win.

Chapter 7
The Velorution

It's suspicious when GW authorities routinely advise consumers to change their light bulbs to reduce GHG. Like that will really help.   Screw in a mercury dusted fluorescent bulb made in China with coal powered energy. Residential lighting is a token cause of GHG production. Commercial lighting burns way more juice, but is more than 90% fluorescent already. Reducing residential lights wattage, sheer numbers and turning them off when not in use, will save money and more GHG than buying more efficient ones, considering the energy used by Americans to earn money and drive to a big box store for new lights.

Ironically the electricity saved by this consumer screwing is compared to the number of cars taken off the road.   Motor vehicles, not light bulbs, are a major cause of GHG in the U.S., but incandescent light bulbs are targeted instead of SUV's.

Transportation produces 34% of GHG in the US. Cars and light trucks use 9 million barrels of oil a day, larger trucks use 2.5 million barrels, airplanes burn through 1.2 million, ships and boats consume 0,7, and railroad trains use 0.3 million barrels. The EPA estimated that vehicles could increase fuel efficiency 80% over the next fifty years. New efficient jets jam-packed with passengers are half as carbon intensive as single passenger cars driving the same distance. But because their GHG is emitted at high altitudes they cause twice as much heat retention.

Forty four percent of national emissions of GHG are from residential and commercial buildings, including lighting, but our vehicles are the major source. In California, transportation accounts for 60% of CO2 emissions, with motor vehicles emitting 94% of this. In Marin County, California, 70% is from single passenger vehicles, since there's little manufacturing, electricity generation, industrial agriculture, air, rail or shipping transport while heating and cooling needs are lower than buildings farther inland, south or north.

The average suburban/exurban Marinade has a carbon footprint twice the size of someone in Brooklyn from driving farther from separate residences that require far more energy and resources than denser neighborhoods in smaller apartments in shared structures. The Good Life in the Suburbs comes with an unsustainable embedded energy cost and those who enjoy it will defend it until collapse. Marin County's daily newspaper, the Marin Independent Journal has been printing irate letters for the last two years about the "monstrosity" or "abomination" of a four story apartment complex going up adjacent to Highway 101. It's not even "affordable" housing, just not as unaffordable as most houses in Marin. The horror, the horror.

AWOL is dependent on motor vehicles. An entire lifestyle evolved from traffic being given priority over people after WWII, when most roads and newer suburban communities were designed and built. Bicyclists lobbied for the first asphalt-paved roads in their brief decades of glory around 1900, but soon the Motorist was King. Mr. Toad's Wild Ride symbolized the priority of the horseless carriage.

The first motorcars were owned by the upper crust, the first trucking companies by industrialists extracting profits from public roads. Ninety percent of public funding for transportation in the twentieth century went to building and maintaining highways for unfettered use of private vehicles. The rest went to mass transit, mainly buses and rail boondoggles. For over a century we've poured 99% of ground transportation resources into the infrastructure, enforcement, supplies and privileges of road hogging motor vehicles.

Electric trolleys morphed into diesel buses and interstate highways became private "freeways" for cars. In suburban and exurban communities, people have to drive many miles to work, shop and socialize because of the dangers and distances involved, while all the stuff we consume and throw away is trucked in and out from some other place on those roads.

Transportation planners crafted wider lanes to accommodate "unimpeded flow" for "traffic safety", and to facilitate evacuation and cleanup after a nuclear crisis during the Cold War. Fire departments pushed for major roads wide enough for two fire engines to pass in opposite directions at fifty miles an hour. Wider roads encourage higher speeds causing far more deadly collisions. A major proportion of fire and rescue calls respond to traffic collisions.

Peter Swift studied traffic and fire injuries over eight years in Longmont, Colorado, comparing areas with wide or narrow streets. While there were no deaths or injuries from fires, there were over 200 traffic injuries and ten deaths. His analysis showed that 36' wide streets were four times as dangerous as 24' streets. The San Francisco Fire Department chief is balking at city plans to create pedestrian friendly streets for a new development that are only 26 feet wide.

Those roads with the unfortunate aspect of being designed with wider lanes, expanded clear zone setbacks for "safer" driving at high speed have few pedestrians. Those that also serve as residential and commercial streets are far more dangerous than roads with narrow lanes, closed in by sidewalks, trees, on street parking and cluttered with other users. Drivers use the "safer" highways as if they were limited access freeways, but unexpected interactions with slower and turning motor vehicles, bicycles and pedestrians are frequent and fatalities common. These road designs were and still are the gold standard of "safe" traffic design.

Public roadways plus parking and service areas take up 40% of urban areas and about half that in most suburbs. Most asphalt is black, sucking up solar heat and causing urban island greenhouse bubbles with average temperatures 3-4 degrees higher than nearby countryside. That is an enormous acreage that could generate revenue or provide public benefits as green parks that cool cities and absorb rainfall, instead of draining them into overloaded sewage systems.

Typical GHG reduction plans focus on token gestures like changing light bulbs or alternative fuels. California tried to regulate GHG from motor vehicles, by classifying it as air pollution, but the EPA said it's a national issue, not a state's right. Then Attorney General Jerry Brown took the feds to court over this, now as Governor he's fine with fracking. GHG reduction would result from basing registration fees on vehicle weight, horsepower and top speed.

The federal government is not likely to solve our energy crisis. Cave in on raising vehicle fleet mileage more than token amounts because apparently "Detroit can't build fuel efficient vehicles", then bail them out when gas prices double and Americans buy fewer SUVs and light trucks, then subsidize corn ethanol to produce less fuel than could be conserved when we start buying New Detroit trucks and SUV's again. Obama did force Detroit to close that "light truck" loophole in mandating higher fuel efficiency standards for their fleets, sometime in the next decade.

The answer is not alternatives to fuel our vehicles or more oil, but using far less of it. Reducing the speed limits on all public roads by 5-15 mph, improving mass transit and rewarding ride sharing would save money for individuals and slash oil prices by greatly reducing demand. Driving slower would reduce public costs from medical care for accidents and pollution. Cyclists and pedestrians would feel safer, helping them to lose weight and save even more money.

We're addicted to speeding in our single passenger, motor vehicles. A tiny minority actually drives the posted speed limit, saving 15% on gas. Other drivers curse them with more vehemence than profiteering oil companies, even more than recreational bicyclists for impeding their right to speed.

Trying to enforce lower speed limits with traditional methods is ineffective and expensive. Regulating all vehicle speeds with wireless engine governors would save more GG and public monies than police ticketing and speed humps. We'd sooner drill off every coastline and plow every field for fuel than slow down or get out of our womb with a view.

The only positive spin about making ethanol fuel from corn is that it makes high fructose corn syrup more expensive. This could reduce obesity and diabetes caused by food manufacturers glopping cheap sweetening into every supersized bite. The ethanol scam the feds have been heavily subsidizing turns corn into gas for SUV's. More corn turned into fuel raises prices for animal feed, makes crops worth more, sells tractors and pushes up land values. Every

Presidential candidate has to kiss the Corn King in Iowa by New Year's Eve of election year.

Corn ethanol takes more fossil fuel energy to produce a gallon than it reduces GHG from the tailpipe. Sugar cane, hemp, switch grass and tropical grasses and canes have far more efficient ratios of conversion to ethanol, but it's telling when farming for fuel takes precedent over food and fiber. We can't grow enough fuel for a transportation system dominated by motor vehicles.

Bio-diesel is the most promising alternative fuel since diesel engines are more efficient than gasoline powered, and some plant oils have a higher net energy gain than ethanol. Even so, it is best used as a 5-15% additive to petroleum diesel to significantly reduce toxic pollutants in diesel exhaust. Running all diesel engines entirely on bio-diesel would require clear cutting the last tropical jungles for palm oil plantations, plowing entire plains for GMO canola, and covering desert sands in algae ponds brewing oil to meet current petroleum diesel demand. Using a lot less vehicle fuel has to become our mantra, not coming up with more of it.

Medical costs from Motor Vehicle Traffic (MVT) are mostly shouldered by society. Thirty thousand are killed each year, while every 20 seconds an American is seriously injured in a traffic accident. Medical treatment for victims of MVT accidents consumes significant Emergency Room costs. Traffic accidents are a primary cause of chronic pain for many Americans, who often spiral into pain med addiction.

Adults are twice as likely to die from heart or lung disease when they live near high traffic areas. MVT spews 79% of the particulate pollution and 91% of air related cancer risk in Marin county, CA. Highway noise raises blood pressure and causes sleep disturbance, known to cause weight gain and irritable behavior. Living near highways increases rates of both human and doggie dementia.

If their externalized costs weren't heavily subsidized, gas would cost over $20 a gallon, licensing fees would be tripled, traffic fines quadrupled. Those costs are covered by general funds or debt now. Only parking fees sometimes generate more revenue than expenses, not counting the lost property value from free parking spaces, or the burden on storm drainage/sewer systems from impervious surfaces.

Drivers can do a lot to save money and reduce GHG right now, no matter what kind of vehicle they're driving. Accelerate and decelerate slowly, inflate tires, regular tune-ups, reduce weight and drag. You've heard those tips, maybe even followed them. One thing you'll rarely hear is to simply drive the speed limit. If we all slowed down to posted limits, instead of driving within the normal range of 8-15 mph faster, Americans would save 20% on fuel, with significantly less vehicle maintenance costs and fewer collisions. That would reduce GHG along with fumes, dust, noise and medical costs from MVT. Pedestrians and cyclists would feel safer, instead of startling as motorists blow by.

Transportation Apartheid is prevalent nearly everywhere across America. Where sidewalks are present they're usually narrow, cluttered and rutted. Cyclists are squeezed out to the crumbling edges of the pavement as wider vehicles proliferate. Bus trips typically take twice as long as driving, unless they have a high speed bus only lane and pre-ticket boarding stations. Poorly funded transit is inevitably late when you're on time and on time when you're late, until eventually you're fired for being frequently late.

Road redesign can calm traffic with Complete Streets that are safer and more pleasant for all users. We can purposely design and fund a more pleasant, safe and convenient transportation system to walk, bicycle, rideshare, drive when needed or use convenient and comfortable mass transit while increasing costs and time to drive alone.

Reforming toxic, dangerous, heat absorbing, water repelling asphalt into pervious sidewalks, trees, bus shelters and parklets creates safer streets that reduce flooding. Complete Streets encourage people to walk, bicycle, shop and linger, reducing GHG while creating neighborhoods that are quieter and cleaner with improved property values.

In *Small Houses*, Jay Schafer points out that people feel more comfortable in neighborhoods where roads are no more than twice as wide as its buildings are tall. Three to four stories with setbacks allows solar exposure, shade when needed and limits wind tunneling of taller buildings. The sense of enclosure is aesthetically pleasing and more calming to humans on foot. We feel safer than being exposed as prey on the vast open spaces that highways create.

Sustainable Communities, a 1986 book by Sym Van der Ryn, describes neighborhoods designed to encourage walking. They are an "affirmation of the street, making it more than a corridor for cars, that binds neighborhoods together." When a speeding car killed a Dutch journalist's child, he began an organization called "Stop the Child Murders". With that urgency they forced engineers to create "woonerf" neighborhoods where cars were restricted in speed and priority by planters, surfaces and right angle turns. This has spread across Europe and given rise to pedestrian priority planning. Pedestrian and mass transit users want streets that feel safer from speeders, and are watched over by neighbors and slow motorists. Not surprisingly those neighborhoods have higher property values.

Improving sidewalks and crosswalks is essential for encouraging walking, the most affordable, healthiest, lifetime exercise and community builder available. Americans only walk an average of a quarter mile a day, down from three miles a century ago. If a trip is longer than 400 yards, half of adults will drive rather than walk. Even convenience stores are farther than that in most suburbs, while half of schools are three miles from students' homes. Only one-third of children walk to school, even when they live less than a mile away, because their parents are reasonably afraid of traffic. One reason half of adults and one third of children in America are overweight.

Increasing the comfort and safety of walking for most short trips is essential to lowering medical costs and GHG. Protection from seasonal heat with shade trees will also allow winter sunlight onto wider sidewalks that aren't obstructed, cracked and pitted. Greenhouse enclosed sidewalks in frigid climates, with awnings, canopies, overhangs or trees shading them in hotter ones will enable four-season exercise for transportation. Rubberized surfaces using recycled tires will cushion impact for exercisers and routine falls of elderly and young.

Slowing down traffic, confining loose dogs and providing jobs to deconstruct the roads in urban and poorer neighborhoods will make them safer and more pleasant to walk in. More walkers means more visibility, greater safety, more socializing. Driving the speed limit will Calm Traffic more effectively than a mother with a baby buggy. Driving at speed limits as Pace Cars is a baby step. Drivers curse us, while pedestrians and cyclists cheer us.

Bicycles are the most efficient form of transportation on the planet, but in this country they are mainly dangerous toys, if they're not sitting in a garage with flat tires. The number one reason Americans give for not bicycling is traffic danger, although 90% of cycle injuries are rider only. Sixty percent of bicycle fatalities are from collisions with motor vehicles, however.

A new improved Safety Cycle is the solution. A recumbent tricycle with some load capacity, assisted by a small electric engine with an aerodynamic shell to protect from weather and impacts will get more Americans out of their cars.

Riders will be cushioned in a foam padded, carbon fiber shell. Psychologically they'll feel cocooned in a womb with a view. Being exposed to every distracted, impaired and aggressive motorist can provoke panic attacks. Painful seating is the number two reason people don't ride and aerogel recumbent seats are far more comfortable than leather saddles. Most cyclists hate hills and headwinds too. A battery powered or ethanol fueled micro engine makes any cyclist going up hills a Lance Armstrong without steroids

Traveling more places without needing to get in their gas guzzler would save money, help people lose weight and get fit through human powered mass transit. The CycleTrain! a human powered mass transit system is the mass transit of the future, along with Bicycle Buses. Commuters will pedal or row as part of a super light train of human powered vehicles gliding along on a monorail embedded in the pavement or on the cheapest elevated transit option possible. People Power utilizes available resources to reduce GHG and obesity in America.

Those early adopters will save money, lose weight and feel better about themselves. Paying people for not driving from cap and trade or carbon tax funds will incentivize alternative transportation users. Drive up the costs of driving with carbon taxes and congestion pricing and only the wealthiest will be able to afford it, but unless alternatives are available Americans will still drive after they can't afford to legally.

Changing traffic use habits will require a long-term realignment of funding. This won't be politically popular. Most drivers will complain mightily rather than switch. For most Americans owning an automobile is an economic necessity for AWOL. It's an addiction more powerful than drink, socially sanctioned despite the expense and damage to the General Welfare. Without organized demands, politicians, transportation planners and those who counsel them will favor private vehicles. Few politicians dare to propose reducing subsidies for MVT.

Commercial traffic will be a tougher challenge, but trucks can be far cleaner, quieter and more efficient, even electric hybrids and transport goods on unjammed roads with fewer personal vehicles.

All the talk about sustainability and cutting off our carbon pinky toes means diddly as long as politicians and planners continue pandering to motor vehicles. They have to because we won't elect anyone who doesn't. Right now only the poorest people depend on "alternative" transportation. After this recession, half the country is officially impoverished. Except for the top twenty percent, the rest are struggling to make ends meet. Unless we admit that we're powerless to change our relationship to MVT and take a lot more than twelve steps to do so, we're not going to reduce GHG, lose weight or save money.

Chapter 8
Put the Lime in the Coconut

The US emits 25% of the planet's human generated GHG, mostly from use of fossil fuels by our military, for electricity generation, our buildings and transportation. The dire warnings about impending climate change, even from the military, should have made curtailing our carbon footprint an emergency, but like frogs in heating water we aren't alarmed.

The Health Care system as it's euphemistically called, may generate almost as much GHG as these Fossil Fuel Four. The US funds "Defense" at around $1 Trillion a year, (with hidden costs), more than the next twenty or so nations combined. Americans spent triple that on medical treatment last year. While flow of cash isn't an exact correlation with GHG production, they closely parallel in our fossil fueled economy. Americans aren't getting much value for three trillion dollars, since every other industrial nations spends far less while their citizens enjoy better health by every measure. ObamaCare isn't likely to change that.

Most progressives believe that Single Payer Health Care will fix a broken system, as if funding the mess would solve the myriad health problems plaguing our citizens. It's hard to fathom this confidence, when the Institute of Medicine's own figures blame medical treatment for causing more deaths in the US than anything except heart disease and cancer. An unknown number of those are also caused by medical treatment.

To be sure, significant costs could be saved by reducing 20% administrative overhead of the private insurance industry to the 3% of Medicare/Medicaid or the 1.5% of Canada's national health care agency. Even If we could find enough MDs willing to take M&M patients without committing fraud, it would still cost a fortune without making Americans healthier. Medical doctors don't create health, they treat diseases. If better health results, that's almost an anomaly.

Conventional medicine enjoys a lucrative monopoly on reimbursed "health" care without producing proportionate results. Americans suffer from epidemics of heart disease, cancer, diabetes, asthma, respiratory and autoimmune diseases, depression, motor vehicle and gun trauma, alcoholism, substance abuse, chronic pain, autism, neurological malfunctions, viral and bacterial infections along with a host of other health problems. Not all the fault of modern medicine, but it persists in only treating the symptoms of a sick and toxic society, squandering resources that could fund public health measures to prevent most of these epidemics.

Lifestyle and environmental illnesses can be prevented for a dime on the dollar costs of relying on conventional medical treatment to pick up the disastrous results. It's time to expand the definition of health care to public health measures that promote social changes and individual practices known to create health, not simply treat symptoms. Systemic changes that enable and encourage Americans to develop healthier habits will eradicate and heal more diseases than vaccines and antibiotics ever did. Actually they already did that when public health funding created cleaner water, air and food, eradicating 90% of fatalities from infectious diseases decades before vaccines and antibiotics stole the credit.

Overwhelming evidence proves that if Americans walk regularly, eat more vegetables, stop smoking, drink less, strengthen social ties, live in a more equal society, gain higher education, have a job that pays enough to reduce financial stressors with time for relaxation and recreation will do more to improve our health than single payer medical insurance. A health care system that pursues those attainable goals will truly be a Universal Health Care.

As usual, there are politically powerful and vastly wealthy interests that are solidly opposed to systemic changes that threaten their profits; regardless of how much GHG they reduce. *Save Trillions with Universal Health Care*, the primary book in my Medical Monopoly series, provides a strategic plan for building coalitions that undermine their influence and sap their entrenched positions to gain such a system, It will also reduce our exposure to toxic substances and hazardous practices by charging Medical Expense Fees to pay for their costs, and fund UHC is necessary.

Currently patients who choose most Complementary and Alternative Medical (CAM) treatments pay out of their own pocket, since medical insurance doesn't cover this care, whether effective or not. The American Medical Association doesn't like any competition, calls 'em all quacks. Yet Americans already spend more out of pocket for CAM, than for conventional medicine, including deductibles. ObamaCare considered, then dropped demands for reimbursement only for evidence based medicine because there wasn't that much. A Dartmouth professor and the Institute of Medicine found that $800 billion a year was spent on treatments that did not provide better outcomes than no treatment at all. Many were "proven" by profit driven, medical industry funded, conducted and published studies. Placebos or more affordable alternative treatments should also be reimbursed since evidence based medicine is not required.

Universal Health Care (UHC) that provides Freedom of Choice by paying for treatment by licensed practitioners and certified therapists providing Physical, Psychological, Social and/or Spiritual health care would build coalitions of support for more inclusive health care reform, Paying for more varieties of treatment will actually cost less than funding only conventional care, with better results for many American maladies and less medically induced damages. This would cost less than bailing out billionaires when they crash the economy.

Medical doctors and their associations have been solidly against reimbursing any alternatives to their monopoly for decades, but conventional medicine would still keep a huge chunk of the patient pie. They enjoying prescription privileges for massively advertised pharmaceuticals and are the only game in town for surgical replacement of aging parts. Because patients with chronic illness and those near death are the largest drain on the system, they might accept cheaper alternatives for them if put to the gun.

UHC could realize huge savings from changing treatment goals for the 20% of the population that 80% of medical costs are spent on. These patients have one or more chronic illness or are near death. Most chronic illnesses are almost entirely lifestyle induced, and the natural death process has been manipulated into an expensive, tortuous gauntlet of heroic treatments. However, these patients may be the least likely to want to change current approaches, regardless of expense and ineffectiveness.

Americans can really reduce GHG by shifting from our wasteful, obesity inducing, consumptive lifestyles. Selling UHC as a way to *Lose Weight, Feel Better and Really Reduce GHG* may be more appealing to Americans than saving trillions. Toss in Whiter Teeth, Better Sex and Fewer Fears and we're home free.

Providing Health Care that provides all that will be far more effective at changing behaviors than a guilt tripping environmental Cassandra. Subsidizing health care rebates to Americans who don't own motor vehicles, eat mainly plants, farm organically, develop renewable energy, live in small homes, earn and spend less money, don't practice war no more, etc... might just save the planet.

Implementing Medical Expense Fees (MEF) on known or suspected causes of illness and injury that directly pay for their medical costs is more politically feasible than simply raising taxes for Single Payer options. charging fees for specific products and practices based on their known medical costs will split business opposition to higher taxes on employment. Polluting, Hazardous Industries will be isolated from the growing Green Business, Natural Capitalism models.

It's almost futile to try to ban toxic substances, look at Alcohol, Tobacco. Diesel Exhaust, Radiation or Aspartame. It took a decade to ban DDT after Rachel Carson wrote the bestseller, Silent Spring, and even then manufacturers just shipped it off to the third world. It's still in American mothers' milk. There's 80,000 synthetic chemicals already in play, and 2, 000 new ones added each year, with only a few dozen having been banned or even regulated. Most safety tests are done by the manufacturers, like pharmaceuticals.

There's little economic incentive for government to try to ban health hazards, but charging fees to pay for their costs will reduce their use. Government loves to discover new ways to raise money and there's no shortage of products and practices to charge MEF on. If fees are levied on the Precautionary Principle, when enough evidence indicates a likelihood of harm, we won't have to wait until overwhelming scientific proof emerges that they've been killing people and the environment for decades and will persist for decades more.

Funding from MEF will keep Medicare/Medicaid solvent even through the oncoming silver tsunami that will soon swamp it. Charging for exposing Americans to Greasy, Sweetened, Salted Foods, Inflammatory Agents, Free Radicals, Radioactive Emissions, Fossil Fuel toxins, Heavy Metals, Endocrine Disruptors, Excessive Speed and other products and practices causing Mortality, Illness or Injury will eventually lower medical costs from these.

Chapter 9
The Fall of Western Civ

Agriculture is the basis of what we think of as civilization-cosmopolitan, wealthy, urban complexes with sprawling hinterlands where the food is grown by peasants. No civilization has ever survived extreme climate change, while many have failed because their agricultural and social practices destroyed their local sustainability. The dominance of industrialized agriculture in the 20th century threatens global collapse of civilization from unsustainable practices for the first time.

It used to take shit and sweat to grow food, fiber, fuel and fodder for the castle keep; now oil and natural gas keep it afloat. Burning them and churning them for pesticides, herbicides, fertilizer, irrigation, harvesting, and running machine engines is needed to plant, maintain, harvest and transport farm product to markets.

If you think the government ought to make a law to save western civ, which many prophets claim will fall due to GW, they could start with reducing GHG generated by American agriculture. The Omnibus Farm Bills passed over the last decades took a fleet of diesel buses to carry all the pork they ladled out to American industrial agricultural. Those Farm Bills never reduced GHG from American agriculture, another major source of national GHG production.

Federal pork for agricultural corporations in the alternative fuel bills was supposedly to rescue us from the 'energy crisis' of rising cost and dependence on foreign oil. More greenhouse gases are produced to grow corn for fuel, because more net energy is used than saved from adding ethanol to gasoline. The Gulf of Mexico Dead Zone is fed from corn fertilizer runoff. Our production of food is as heedless of the ecology as zombies eating brains.

Our transportation system is intimately related with the ag industry from non-stop truck delivery of products to supermarkets and drive through dispensers. Being able to see our toes could be the impetus for Americans to reform agriculture and transportation without waiting on the feds to act. Promising citizens that they will Lose Weight and Feel Better while Reducing GHG from agricultural production is more likely to reduce our fossil fuel consumption than predicting civilization-collapsing calamities.

If we ate a plant based, locally grown, organic diet with grass fed meat, pastured eggs and butter we would really reduce GHG, lose weight and save money instead of bankrupting our children's future. Not everyone can afford this, although in the long run no one can afford not to. Industrialized agriculture has managed to reduce the costs of food as a percentage of income for Americans. Non-nutritious food is ludicrously cheap, while organic can seem a bit steep. Housing and transportation gobble up more income the less you earn, but food is comparatively cheap for most classes. Many Americans rely on packaged or fast foods loaded with grease, sweeteners, mystery meats and refined flours for their calories because they seem the cheapest and are purposefully addictive. That's why poorer Americans are the most obese.

Food Stamps, actually food debit cards now, are the biggest subsidy in the Farm Bills. They typically enable poor people to buy processed foods available in their neighborhood bodegas, enriching Big Food companies and Industrial Agriculture. Nutritional Education and enabling food credit users to use them for more affordable, fresher vegetables and fruit, whole grains, greens, and less processed products will be healthier for them and the planet. It will also lower Medicare costs. Cheap calories are pushed on the poor now as their only way to save money, even though lowering costs for housing and transportation would save far more of their income. Financial stress causes obesity, one reason there's more fat, poor people than rich ones. It contributes to insomnia, divorce, abortion, chronic illness and premature death.

All humans on the planet can be fed sufficiently on what is grown right now with leftovers, depending on what we eat. Not how much. We don't need to grow more food to End Hunger. We simply need to eat less meat. GMO's are not going to feed the hungry billions; they're primarily feeding livestock and making fuel. Ten billion humans could feast on nutritious vegan gruel, laced with insect, leaf and algae protein, preferably caffeinated in the morning and sedating in the evening, without damaging the environment.

Americans aren't likely to adopt such a completely balanced, perfectly sustainable diet, until that's all that's left, without some prodding and promoting. The wealthy and educated are increasingly choosing organic, locally grown produce, whole grains, and grass fed protein sources. Pushing public tastes towards foods requiring fewer petroleum inputs, miles to market, and confined feedlots will reduce agriculture's footprint significantly. This shouldn't just be for the well to do. Inner cities and suburbs can sprout Victory Gardens instead of trashed lots and endless lawns.

Organic farming is millennia older than industrial, chemical based farming, which emerged to dominate after WWII. The new farming has used ever more poisons for pests and dumped fossil fuel based fertilizers on sterilized fields to yield monocrops, instead of building soil fertility and plant health with age-old organic practices. The much-maligned hippies championed organic farming after they went back to the land in the 70's. Now it's going corporate after Middle America woke up in the 90's wanting safer, tastier, more environmentally benign food. The higher prices commanded by organic produce supported the ability of smaller, local farmers to earn a living. That's in danger from demands to bastardize federal organic standards, consolidation and market pressure for lower wholesale prices, rising living costs for farmers and outright cheating by ag and food corporations to capitalize on the growing demand for organic.

The next microniche for sustaining small farmers will be practicing biodynamic, permaculture and agro-agriculture principles of farming. These innovative systems heal the land instead of extracting and poisoning, utilize natural materials and protections to control pests. They have far smaller carbon footprints than industrial organic farming, which is far smaller than conventional. The Farm Bill could have switched allegiance from chemicalized, industrial Ag corporations to whole heartedly supporting small scale, localized, organic and beyond agriculture producers, researchers, inspectors and consumers. That would have made a huge dent in America's

GHG production from agriculture and our poor health. Our fearless leaders choose to talk about change, without doing much to push for it.

We're living the Vida Loco with our diet, which depends on Big Ag, a fundamental base for the wasteful, obesity inducing, debt loaded AWOL. It isn't making us happy; we're putting on weight, spending our children's inheritance, and changing the climate to feed our addictions. We're probably going to need an intervention to give up our wasteful use of fossil fuels, however bleak predictions of impending doom only breed despair. Don't Panic, Go Organic.

Chapter 10
Flickering Blue Tubes

Two devices emblematic of AWOL increase GHG and obesity. Both are shiny and fast, at least when new, and addictive to the extreme. Automobiles and televisions (now electronic screens) embody AWOL, which is both greenhouses gassy and extra wide. Televisions and electronic hardware use 20% of the electricity in some households. BlueRay wide screens vampire electricity even when they're off. These wipe out any reductions from changing light bulbs.

The massive servers receiving, storing, and transmitting all those bits and bytes of electrons require less electricity than forging steel and iron, but they aren't carbon neutral. Ginormous server buildings that rely on cooling their processors with fans use about 2% of U.S. energy and almost as much water as fracking. This is forecast to quadruple by 2020. Our online connectedness requires a hefty amount of energy for servers and processors that can be reduced by burying them in the far north. There they will probably be powered by tar sands and oil extracted from the melting arctic, if we don't reduce our demands for energy.

There are over one billion PC's and two billion televisions on the planet now. Television also generates GHG by churning desires for shiny large vehicles to chase the glamorous lifestyles and starter castles shown on screen. Hollywood generates more GHG by spreading the glory of AWOL to developing nations. Their elite emulate this lifestyle, while their poor desire it, fast cars, big homes, guns and all. Even the colossal amounts of CO_2 Hollywood has spewed producing moving images for consumption, will be dwarfed if everyone adopts the unsustainable lifestyle they portray.

While watching TV generates fewer GHG than driving, both cause extra weight gain. Each strains reality through a glass screen, like a womb with a view. Neither requires much physical energy from the user, although falling asleep while watching the tube is generally less hazardous than while driving.

Watching TV and driving fast generates endorphins, a brain chemical indicted in most addictive activities. It makes us feel better just by taking us out of our negative thought patterns for a spell. But it's not relaxing for our bodies. People watching a show or driving are physiologically stimulated without physically releasing tension, aroused without gaining the relief of fight or flight movement.

Paralyzed in the helpless prey pose the fight instinct rapidly comes into play for frustrated drivers. Television viewers are more heavily sedated, unless they're yelling at Fox TV or NFL football. Most merely nod their heads to the burning bush reciting modern commandments on what to think about, desire and buy.

Americans could give up their televisions without social consequences today, if not their smart phones. The more time people spend glued to an electronic screen the more likely they are to be overweight, lonely, depressed, envious, slothful, gluttonous and several other deadly sins along with life threatening medical conditions. There are health costs just from carrying these EMF emitters close to your body. The reinforcement of negative emotions, violent actions and dystopian culture that entertainment and news focuses on is even more sickening. This self-imprisonment in a culturally reinforced belief system is more difficult to escape than taking the red or blue pill in *The Matrix*.

Television and computers are symbolic of the electron driven third industrial revolution, which began at the end of WWII with the explosion of the atomic bomb. Computers were born out of that cauldron as well, emerging from the artillery tabulators and cryptographic decoders of the First World War. Every new Industrial Revolution has been followed by a social revolution, but the information revolution is creating a connected and surveilled society to tamp down any social unrest, for our own good, of course.

The social disruptions careening in the wake of previous technological shifts were anti-authoritarian and democratic in nature. The authorities are doing their utmost to keep society chained to their screens, limited to "liking" democratic and equalizing memes. Turning the armada of military space satellites into global communication cells for real Freedom of

Speech will symbolize that they did not succeed. With geosynchronous orbits, these transformed military weapons and spy satellites will transmit open sourced, transparent and positive solutions to the planetary crisis. No more cell towers over playgrounds, posing as pine trees.

This citizen revolution requires a commitment to alternative choices of entertainment and some will power at first. Will power is easier to exercise when we associate an undesirable action with a negative reaction that outweighs any short-term benefits. Paying attention to the effect on our affect of watching screens for too long is the first step. AWOL is horrible for our health, but we don't seem to have enough energy to snap out of it without the blue pill. Or was that the red one? Our memories dissipate under attack from EMF waves. We're stuck in the web of "everyone else is doing it." Our mothers once asked whether we'd BASE jump off a cliff if everyone else did it. We're approaching the edge.

Chapter 11
A Better Future Being Born

At least two distinctly different futures are possible for the USA, based on our energy choices. Stay the course and slide into a dystopian nightmare. A toxic wasteland nation where the wealthiest are sheltered along with their myriad servants in undisclosed locations, while the masses survive in mean poverty or increasingly desperate striving to maintain AWOL.

Since this dystopian future requires no real change, it's favored by inertia. However a growing chorus of warming frogs clamors for an insanely industrial society to rapidly switch to renewable resources and intense conservation of non-renewable ones. This future means a healthier, safer, more egalitarian country, favoring the General Welfare over the Common Defense. The Hydra headed Military Complex will have to be slashed back repeatedly to birth this future. That rough beast alone could kill it in its crib. Fossil fueled interests cursed this infant at its christening.

Few experts give this sapling of a future much chance, but Americans have rallied resiliently when faced with extreme challenges. We believe in Progress, it's our true national religion. We've been sold a bill of goods that progress means only economic gain, but a cleaner, safer, healthier, thriftier, regenerative and egalitarian society is true progress.

There's a multitude of prophets preaching the Green Gospel of a New Wine. That another Great Awakening in our history will guide us to adopting Lifestyles Of Health and Sustainability (LOHAS). Our Hopes for a Better World and Desire for Real Change will bear fruit when we elbow our "leaders" out of the way, because they are bought and sold in the marketplace.

The Paley Commission reported back to Democrat President Truman in 1952, recommending America develop renewable resources to create prosperity. It predicted a solar future by 1975. A year later, Republican Eisenhower tossed it aside for the military industrial complex and the "Peaceful

Atom". Nuclear power would be "too cheap to meter". After a half trillion was sunk into "the most expensive technological failure in human history", no new plants were built after 1974.

Jimmy Carter, Democrat put solar hot water panels on the White House and started the national Solar Energy Research Institute. He also managed to make conservation look like sacrifice instead of a virtue, and spent billions on a disastrous Shale Oil boondoggle.

Reagan tore the panels down and pimped for petroleum. The Oiliest President, Poppy Bush, brought most of the world into his Gulf War for Oil. In the waning days of Clinton's administration, the National Renewable Energy Laboratory confirmed that all of the electricity used by the US could be generated with renewables by 2020. Then another crude oiled Bush with tarred and chickenhawk feathered Cheney left us mired in the tar sands of empire, trading blood for oil disruption.

Solartopia by Harvey Wasserman, spins a Green Fantasy of how we get from here to 2030, without cooking the climate, nuking the planet or devolving into shantytowns burning libraries to stay warm. Developing decentralized small scale wind, biomass, geothermal, hydro and solar power along with Co-generation ocean platforms, super efficient buildings and machines may not fuel the current industrial society, but we can re-create it as healthier, quieter, cleaner, safer and sustainable one with a practical vision and supportive policies. Humans are not necessarily a plague on the environment, although we've chosen that option for a few millennia.

Cities are reborn as energy and food producing vertical gardens using their own waste to make compost and natural gas. Renewable resources are owned by the public like the four wind turbines built in Ohio in 2004-5. Wasserman forecasts "Windiana", when the Great Lakes and Great Plains have sprouted more community owned turbines than corn silos. Corn based ethanol was phased out in favor or waste based, while hybrid motor vehicles use much less gas.

A reliable, efficient mass transit system is human powered with cycle trains on monorails and bicycle buses. Replacing toxic petroleum with hydrogen, electric or bio-fuels, to move humans in a half-ton beast is shifting chairs on the

Titanic. Besides, routine exercise from commuting will lower medical costs by trillions. A sustainable future is possible, essential even, but getting there from here will be nigh impossible, considering the implacable opposition of Coal, Oil, Nuclear and Gas interests. Wasserman calls them King CONG. With their enormous wealth, influence and ruthless tyranny we are going to need the luck of the Irish, perhaps even luckier, considering their history.

There are many explanatory books, videos and hands on workshops about building a bridge to a Greener Future. It is possible with current technology and practices to create a healthier, more equitably distributed and much wiser society.

We're gonna need to do a lot more than tap our heels three times to flee the clutches of King KONG on COCAINE, aligned with the Military/Industrial complex arrayed against Solartopia, Ecotopia, Paradise Gained. The future vision they offer is more of the same, but worse. The Laws of Inertia predict certain catastrophe. An vision that guarantees Americans they will Lose Weight, Feel Better, Save Money and Really, Reduce Greenhouse Gases can save the planet.

The plant a tree to become carbon neutral will become a giant farce without understanding what trees should be planted where and how to protect a forest by allowing peasants to make a sustainable living in it. Saving existing forests from lumbering and slash/burning is more critical than planting new ones. Millions of the right trees planted in the right place will store carbon for centuries, if they're not logged or burned. Enriching grasslands with compost will store almost as much carbon in the soil, where it can't be burnt only plowed. Grass fed, pastured animals reduce GHG, especially if we eat fewer of them.

In the fine print, sequestering or storing carbon credits can be given for asphalt paving. Build a new road, balance the carbon burned by the motor vehicles with stored petrochemicals in the surface. A ship captain with a load of rust was already planning to trade it for carbon credits, by dumping it in the south Pacific to stimulate plankton growth. He was arrested, but without wise guidance all kinds of crackpot schemes and boondoggles will be hatched.

Reducing global GHG depends on emerging countries choosing more sustainable models, not just industrialized countries. China emits almost 80% of its GHG from industrial processes, making cheaper stuff that Americans buy at Big Box Stores. Assisting less developed nations in leapfrogging the infrastructure built up and discarded during developed nations evolution will steer them away from AWOL. That would reduce more GHG as carbon credits than planting Eucalyptus forests in Africa.

Human powered transportation, construction methods using local and abundant materials, solar or super efficient wood stoves for cooking, space and water heating, composting toilets, bio-intensive gardens, photovoltaic for night lights and digital transmission, low speed wind and water mills for electricity could transform their lives into extremely low GHG emitters, as could retrofitting ours.

For our own health and the resilience of our society, we're going to have to shed our media blinders and idealization of a greasy, sickly, super sized AWOL, instead of a thrifty, lean and healthy lifestyle. The richer tend to be thinner to an unhealthy extreme, ever since the plump plutocrat went out of style. Greater equality through wealth and luxury taxes could reduce obesity among the poor, faster than green coffee extract.

The richest 1% emit more GHG than the bottom 4/5ths of Americans, The managerial class that makes up most of the top quintile is lean compared to the Davos Crowd when it comes to carbon footprints. From their green palaces, jet set travel, pricy entertainment, to their imported luxury items they spew carbon. Calculating the damage done from their income sources and their investment streams requires a super chilled mainframe.

They have more wealth than several billion of the poorest on the planet. Some peasants are so poor they rely on chopping and burning down rainforest for fuel or to sell charcoal for a few pennies. They poach endangered species and graze goats until desertification. Rocket stoves that use twigs to burn super hot without smoke, solar lights and cell phones, composting toilets, permaculture training, camel livestock, leguminous plants, multi-use trees and fog water accumulators are affordable options that could transform the lives of the worlds poorest. Taxing the rich sufficiently to reduce the wealth inequality that is a major generator of GHG will not be easy. In the untied states, the wealthy are revered as if gold glittered deities, given as much free speech as they can buy. Taking them down a peg or two to save the planet has a nice ring, but it will need a social revolution to do so.

This book is my prophetic gift to the people who have read this far.   We can massively reduce GHG. It may not stop GW but it will make us leaner, smarter and sexier. If we don't follow Plan A, we probably won't implement Plan B or C in time either. Plan B mitigation plans might save coastal residents from rising seas threatening their waterfront homes, but Plan C will save trailer trash from EWP. Catastrophic Change favors the Lucky. We've been brainwashed to shop til you drop and believe that whoever dies with the most toys wins. NASCAR Americans may never come round to changing their unsustainable lifestyle because of GW. They might do so to save money and lose weight.

Yes, we should develop appropriate wind, hydro, solar, bio-fuel resources, but beware government backing these alternatives with rhetoric, while actual funding gets dwarfed by corporate giveaways. Vote Religiously, it's not that Hard. Write Letters to the Editor and Walk Your Talk. At least you'll be able to say I Told You So.